DEDICATION

*I dedicate this book to all the health-seeking people who have made
the decision to value their Health*

Contents

What is all the Fuss about Aloe Vera?

Folklore attributes a number of healing properties to a spiky green plant the world today recognizes as aloe vera. Its journey from a folk remedy for quick relief from small burns and cuts to a hero ingredient in health and dietary supplements and beauty aids is nothing short of spectacular. Aloe vera has truly captured the imagination of the health and beauty industry as well as the health- and beauty-conscious consumer. So, why so much fuss about this humble decorative houseplant? To understand this, let's travel back in time from the millennium to BC.

Aloe Vera's status is through the roof!

•   Egyptians queen Cleopatra and Nefertiti use aloe vera extracts in their beauty regimen.

•   Arabs use powdered aloe vera as their go-to medication for a range of external and internal disorders.

•   Alexander the Great authorizes a war just to acquire aloe vera plantations so the plant can be used to continuously heal his wounded soldiers.

•   Hindu and Chinese medics call aloe vera a 'silent healer', and use it extensively in their therapeutic remedies, notably for sinusitis, skin abnormalities and seizures in children.

•   The Knights Templar create an elixir from aloe vera pulp and other ingredients, which they believe can enhance strength and longevity.

Aloe vera's array of medicinal and beauty benefits earned it the moniker of 'miracle plant'. Famous physicians Dioscorides, Pliny the Elder, Gallen, Aretacus and Antyllus expound the benefits of aloe vera in their written works and treatises. They, however, warn that only high-quality and pure aloe vera extracts and products can deliver the efficacy and potency desired of them. Read more in *Chapter 3 'The 4,000 Year History of Aloe Vera'.*

Wait a Minute, isn't all this just Folklore?

Folklore has served up a lot of research material for scientists on a quest to discover new medicines. All folk medicine must face the test of time to become relevant or at least worthy of consideration in the modern Allopathic landscape. Aloe vera is one of the very few to have stood the test of time, proven its effectiveness and provided satisfaction to users. The plant's powerful biochemical properties couldn't be denied; however, evidence of consistent performance was necessary for mass acceptance, and here is where aloe vera faltered a bit.

In the 16th and 17th centuries, countries that imported aloe vera failed to show the same degree of healing as countries where the plant grew naturally and available fresh for use. As I mentioned above, ancient physicians stressed the importance of using quality aloe vera for the plant to work its magic. Balms and medications that didn't use fresh aloe vera leaves were ineffective, and people in Europe and North America rejected the plant's benefits as just folklore. Aloe vera's reputation remained untarnished in South and Central America, as well as the Caribbean.

Resurgence and Present Avatar

In the years that followed, scientists made new discoveries about aloe vera and used advanced techniques that prevented the nutrients and active ingredients in the plant from getting destroyed during extraction.

The evolution of complementary and alternative medicine in the millennium further bolstered the visibility and potential of aloe vera. Today, aloe vera has become a multi-million dollar industry and the subject of laboratory tests to expand on the scientific evidence that can help make the plant more mainstream then its current existence.

Understanding Aloe Vera

Aloe vera is a succulent plant with a northern African origin. It belongs to the Lily family, but looks like a cactus. A species of Aloe (there are between 200 to 400 of them), aloe vera can either be stemless or have short stems. The plant is known for its thick, fleshy, green leaves. These leaves, which can also be gray-green in color, have flecks or tiny thorns on the surface. The plant is recognized world over for its medicinal properties. It may grow between 60 and 100 centimeters.

Aloe vera spreads by its root sprouts and offsets. It grows in a bunch. The houseplant grows in dry and warm climates. Aloe vera plants have the ability to retain moisture by closing their pores. While other plants wilt and die gradually, aloe vera with its moisture-locking properties manages to stay moist even when it does not get enough water. Flowers grow on the plant around summer time. Aloe vera flowers can grow up to 90 cm and have a yellow coloured tubular corolla.

Leaf structure

The gel-filled leaves contain four layers; namely the rind, sap, mucilage gel and aloe vera gel. The rind on the outer layer protects the plant. Did you ever cut an aloe vera leaf and notice a sticky yellowish fluid oozing out of it? It is sap, which is a bitter tasting fluid that forms an extra layer of protection, preventing animals from eating the plant. The mucilage gel, which is found in the center, makes up the inner part of the plant's leaf. Finally, you have the aloe vera gel, resting inside the leaf, under these protective layers. The gel, in its raw form can taste unpleasant due to the bitter sap covering it.

The leaf of the plant is hard and thick (it has a thickness of close to 15 cell layers). It also has a waxy surface, which is due to the high content of calcium and magnesium found in the leaf. Aloe juice is stored inside the thin, long tubes of either phloem or xylem. These tubes are responsible for transporting nutrients and water to the plant. The sap comes out of these large tubes every time an aloe vera leaf is cut.

Many people assume that aloe vera gel and juice are the same thing, but it is not true. Aloe vera gel is what you find inside the leaf, while the juice is the bitter substance under the leaf's skin. Aloe vera juice is also called aloe latex.

Nutritional Value of Aloe Vera

Aloe vera is called a natural healer due to its medicinal properties, which it derives from its components. It contains up to 200 active components. Though aloe vera is 99 percent water, it does contain over 75 known ingredients that make it anti-biotic, anti-bacterial, anti-fungal and anti-septic in nature. Among the most important nutrients found in aloe vera are lignins, saponins, minerals, vitamins, amino acids, enzymes, fatty acids and sugars.

We will have a detailed look at these components and their properties in the next chapter.

The 4,000 Year History of Aloe Vera

Do you remember the first time you were introduced to aloe vera and its list of benefits? Were you told about the 'miraculous' properties of aloe vera by a friend or family member? Or did you stumble upon its rich history on the Internet? Irrespective of when you found out about the therapeutic properties of aloe vera, the wonder plant has been helping generations of humans lead a healthy life for thousands of years now.

Aloe vera, available today in the market in almost every form – be it gels, drinks, pastes or creams - has its origin in the mysterious land of Africa, from where it was soon taken all over the globe, starting with the Middle East and Mediterranean regions.

There is a quite some debate over the origin of this miracle plant, though. Some researchers and historians claim that the plant originated in Africa, while some believe that it was first found in the Arabian region. Then there is another set of historians who are of the opinion that the earliest records of the origin of the plant have been found in Egypt. They believe that aloe vera's antiquity, dating back to 1550 BC, was first discovered in Egypt in 1862.

However, almost every part of the continent has some historic record claiming its years of dependence on aloe vera. In Egypt, it showed up in the form of pictures on walls of religious structures, while there have been references to the plant and its magical powers in Chinese as well as Indian literature. The Sumerian tablet from 2100 BC is one of the oldest records of aloe vera and its recognition by humans. The Bible, too, has references of the Aloes.

However, today the plant is widely grown in almost all parts of the world. Aloe vera is now available in several forms for various medicinal & therapeutic reasons – be it skin care, health care and much more. Wouldn't it be interesting to find out how our ancestors found out about the healing properties of aloe vera and how they used the plant? Then let's go back to the 4th century, where it all started!

How Kings, Queens and Physicians used Aloe Vera in Ancient History

The island of Socotra, quickly became famous in 500 BC for its aloe vera plantations, where the crop was also used to trade with countries like China, India and Tibet. When Aristotle learned about this 'silent healer' as the Indians called it, he informed Alexander The Great about it, and persuaded him to take over the isle so that they could use the plant to heal their soldiers.

In Egypt, aloe vera was given more of a god-like status due to its healing properties. They called it the 'Plant of Immortality'. It was also widely used by the queens of Egypt to enhance their beauty. Cleopatra and Nefertiti, known for their ageless beauty, are believed to have used aloe vera to make their skin look glowing and young. The Mahometans of Egypt also considered aloe vera a religious symbol. They believed it to be a protector that could ward off evil. Aloes were so important for Egyptians back in the ancient times, that it was used as a means to measure a man's wealth.

A physician, who later became the Emperor of Rome, Galen (AD 131-201), gained knowledge about aloe vera and its healing properties. He then used it to treat several wounded Roman soldiers. He authored more than 100 books about natural medicines and their uses, aloe vera being one of them.

Just like Egypt, in Mesopotamia, too, people assumed that aloe vera had the power to protect from evil. They relied on the plant to keep them protected from evil spirits. The Knights of Templar also created an elixir using aloe vera extracts, which they believed increased longevity. It was named the 'Elixir of Jerusalem'.

The Arabs too have a special place for Aloes in their history. They found out that the gel inside the leaf could be separated and used for a variety of purposes. They got the gel by crushing the leaves with their bare feet. They would then cover the crushed pulp with goatskin bags and leave them to dry before making a powder of it. They named the plant 'Desert Lily'.

Aloe vera also impressed King Solomon (971-931 BC) with its multi-benefits. He was so impressed by the plant and the number of ways it could be used that he is said to have employed it for his wedding decoration too.

Pedanius Dioscorides was a Greek physician, botanist and pharmacologist. He wrote about aloe vera and its healing properties in De Materia Medica, an encyclopedia of medicines and herbs. He explained how the plant could be used for treating boils, skin irritations, dental problems, bruises and to hydrate dry skin.

Aloe vera was known as the 'Elixir of Longevity' in Russia, while in China, people have been long known to rely on aloe vera juice to treat rashes. Doctors in China even called it a 'harmonic remedy' when they found out about its medicinal properties.

By 1930s, medical reports started coming out about aloe vera and its medicinal properties. It began with the successful treatment of radium and X-ray burns by using aloe vera. Prior to that, there were instances when aloe vera was used to treat stasis and radiation ulcers. Several case studies and reports have also been found supporting the use of aloe vera to treat frostbites and injuries in animals. Today, aloe vera can be used for almost anything from soothing the skin to managing the treatment of diabetes.

The Health Benefits of Aloe Vera

Aloe vera is known as the plant of immortality, yes. However, it is not just one component that makes it the purest gift from nature. This miraculous plant has been used by humans for its therapeutic effects for more than 5000 years now. The colorless gel in aloe vera is up to 99 percent water, but the plant contains more than 200 active components! No wonder it offers an almost unending list of benefits.

Did you know the gel of the plant contains up to twenty amino acids, eight of which humans cannot create on their own, but need for their existence? Apart from amino acids, aloe vera is also rich in fatty acids including HCL, B-sitosterol, campesterol, myristic, oleic and stearic. Aloe vera is also loaded with vitamins like vitamin A, vitamin C, vitamin E, vitamin B1, B2, B3, B6 and vitamin B12 (one of the few plants to contain it). It is composed of close to 20 minerals, such as sodium, potassium, calcium, zinc, magnesium, copper, chromium and manganese.

Next come the enzymes. These biochemical catalysts break down proteins into amino acids. Among the main enzymes found in aloe vera are bradykinase, cellulase, lipase, oxidase, creatine phosphokinase and alkaline phosphatase. These enzymes break down food in our body, into fuel that can be used by every cell to work efficiently.

Aloe vera also contains a high amount of lignins, which gives the plant its absorbing properties. The miracle plant can penetrate up to seven layers inside the skin, making it highly effective against skin problems. Lignins even break through the most hardened skin.

Apart from fatty acids, amino acids, minerals and vitamins, aloe vera is also known for its sugar content. The sugar chains in the plant fall under the mucopolysaccharides category, which are healthy for the body. Aloe vera also contains saponins, salicylic acid and anthraquinones, which gives the plant its medicinal and healing properties.

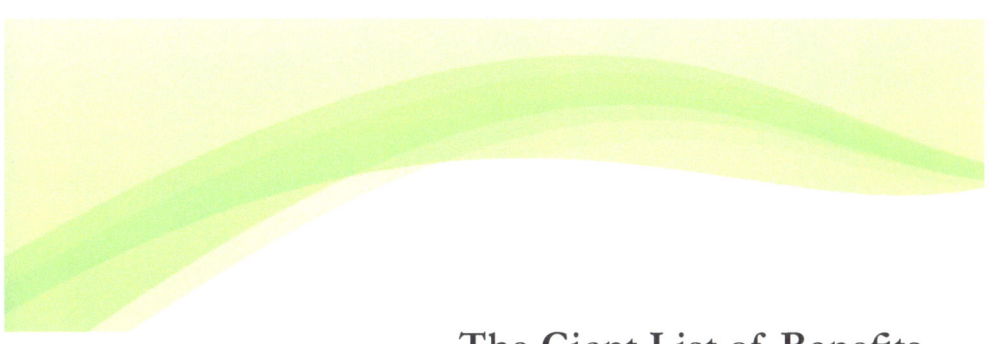

The Giant List of Benefits

Now that you know about the different components that make aloe vera a useful plant in almost every aspect, let's have a look at the ways in which it is useful to the body in detail:

Aloe vera alkalizes the body

Are you aware of the 80/20 rule for great health? It refers to the intake of 80 percent of food that is alkali while consuming only 20 percent that is acidic. However, most people tend to have a diet that is heavier on the acidic side, thereby leading to health complications. Consumption of aloe vera helps alkalize the body, ensuring germs will find it difficult to grow in such an environment. Aloe vera helps balance the acidic content in the body. Its alkaline nature helps maintain the PH level in the body. In addition to it, aloe vera also aids in detoxifying the body and making it toxin-free. In fact, there is a widely popular diet called the 'green diet', which includes the intake of green vegetable supplements and aloe vera juice to help detoxify the body.

Aloe vera keeps dental problems at bay

Aloe vera has been linked with treating a variety of problems relating to teeth and gums. Aloe vera's disinfecting properties make it effective in keeping your mouth protected from dental problems like infections and plaque build-up. Gingivitis is a major and common dental problem that leads to inflammation in the gums. It begins with the build-up of plaque, resulting in gum swelling and even bleeding.

Not only is it painful, gingivitis also puts you at risk of tooth decay. In some cases, the condition can even affect the bones supporting your teeth, putting your whole dental structure at risk. However, using dental products containing aloe vera or oral consumption of the plants gel kills gingivitis-causing bacteria before they can cause any major harm. It prevents plaque build-up, and keeps your teeth germ-free. Aloe vera also comes in handy as a breath freshener, as it keeps your oral cavity protected, which is usually linked with bad breath.

Aloe vera boosts your cardiovascular health

The Journal of Nutritional Science & Vitaminology did a study on the effects of aloe vera consumption on the human body. As per the report, intake of aloe led to a decrease in the cholesterol production in liver by close to 30 percent. Aloe vera juice has also proven useful in keeping a balance between the good and bad cholesterol in the body. It reduces the amount of bad cholesterol in the body, also known as low density lipoprotein (LDL), while increasing the volume of good cholesterol, called high density lipoprotein (HDL). There are a few other natural remedies that help reduce the level of bad cholesterol in the body. However, what makes aloe vera a better choice is that not many natural treatments also help in boosting the level of HDL in the body.

Another major study on aloe vera (conducted over a five-year period), included up to 5000 heart patients. Their health conditions were studied during this period, where they were told to consume bread along with aloe vera twice a day during lunch and dinner. The study showed impressive results when over 90 percent of the participants showed an improvement in their triglyceride, blood sugar and cholesterol levels. The most noticeable result of the study was that none of the 5000 participants suffered another heart attack while following the diet. During this period, they were also asked to refrain from smoking and consuming alcohol.

Aloe vera reduces inflammation

Aloe vera is well known for its anti-inflammatory properties, which it gets from the enzymes in it, namely the pain-fighting bradykinase. Inflammation can affect any part of the body. Fortunately, you can use aloe vera to treat it almost anywhere. Inflammation shows up in the form of swelling, redness, or pain, however, it does not always show on the outside of the body, sometimes it can be internal. This is the body's way of reacting to any infection or injury, so it essential for the body to stimulate immune system defenses and quickly heal from an irritation or injury. However, as it can be painful, you can use aloe vera (either orally or topically) to heal and soothe the inflamed area with the help of salicylic acid, an aspirin-like compound that disrupts the production of prostaglandin hormones, which cause inflammation.

Bradykinase boosts the blood flow in the inflamed area, helping it heal faster, while campesterol (also in aloe vera) helps in the creation of new cells to further contribute to the healing process.

Aloe Vera aids in digestion

The healing properties of the wonder plant are not hidden from many. However, what most people do not know is that aloe vera also helps with digestion. The digestive tract functions by absorbing all the nutrients from food. However, your digestive tract's ability to separate nutrients from the toxins in the food also depends on what kind of diet you follow. If your diet is not healthy, your digestive system may not be able to clean up all the toxins in your tract, thereby leading to their build up. It may lead to irritable bowel syndrome (IBS), when the toxins reaching your colon. It prevents your body from getting nutrients from food, as your blood stream is not able to absorb them. This results in fatigue or malnutrition, before leading to major health issues.

However, aloe vera helps in keeping the digestive system clean and functioning properly by ensuring that food residue and toxins do no clog the tract. Additionally, it can even aid in getting rid of intestinal worms.

Aloe vera boosts the immune system

If your immune system is strong, it will help you stay protected from infections and disease. Your body will heal on its own if your immune system is healthy. However, that is not always the case. From irregular sleeping habits to tiredness (or other aspects of an unhealthy lifestyle), several factors can weaken your immune system over time. In fact, your body can show signs of a weak immune system in the form of constant headaches, forgetfulness, fatigue and stiff joints.

Aloe vera can help you by boosting your immune system and keeping you protected against a large number of diseases. The juice of aloe vera contains polysaccharides, which has a direct and positive effect on the white blood cells in your body. These white blood cells are the ones which bravely fight the viruses trying to make you unhealthy! Aloe vera is rich in antioxidants, further helping you combat unstable compounds (also called free-radicals). These radicals are the ones responsible for making you appear older! Isn't it great how the regular intake of aloe vera can not only keep you healthy, but also looking younger? It is called the miracle plant for a reason (in this case, plenty of reasons)!

Aloe Vera improves blood circulation

You already know how aloe vera boosts your cardiovascular health. Aloe vera is among the few natural (highly effective) options that reduce blood clots in the body. The miraculous plant not only improves the circulation of blood in the body, but also purifies it. Drinking aloe vera juice regularly aids in blood circulation throughout the body as the juice expands the size of blood capillaries, thereby resulting in better and easier circulation. It means your heart gets a healthy supply of fresh blood, which keeps it pumping normally.

By purifying the blood that flows in your body, your internal organs benefit from a greater supply of oxygen too, which improves their functionality. Your body's vital organs like your heart and brain constantly need fresh blood supplied to them, and aloe vera does just that when it purifies your blood. Improves blood circulation also helps with other health conditions like cold toes and fingers and exhaustion (both physical and mental).

Aloe vera balances blood sugar

Did you know that aloe vera helps in the production of insulin as it supports the function of the pancreas? It means the intake of aloe vera can have an effect on your blood sugar level. Is it true though? Has it been proven? The good news is yes, studies have proven that aloe vera juice helps in lowering blood sugar levels.

Compounds like mannans, lectins and anthraquinones present in aloe vera, giving it anti-diabetic properties, make it an effective tool in bringing down glucose levels. Regular intake of aloe vera juice is often suggested to those having diabetes, as well as those who are at the risk of developing it.

Aloe vera juice reduces the amount of blood lipids in diabetics (who usually produce these fats in high amounts). It also has the same effect on those diagnosed with acute hepatitis. Another way in which diabetics benefit from aloe vera intake is with faster healing of wounds and reduced swelling. You already know about the healing and anti-inflammatory properties of aloe vera. Diabetics regularly complain about ulcers and leg injuries. Aloe vera can help diabetics in speeding up the healing process.

Though aloe vera helps greatly in managing diabetes, those who have already been diagnosed with the disease should consult their doctors before introducing aloe vera in their diet or relying on it too heavily. Doctors often advise their patients to drink aloe vera juice before or after meals.

Aloe vera has disinfectant, anti-biotic, anti-microbial, germicidal, anti-bacterial, anti-septic, anti-fungal and anti-viral properties

Whooaa, that's a lot of goodness in just one plant, right? That's what makes aloe vera an effective remedy in almost everything – no matter what your health condition is. Aloe vera is among the oldest and widely used anti-biotic and anti-bacterial plants. Its anti-bacterial properties provide protection against infections (usually caused by viruses, bacteria and fungi). It is a major ingredient in several antiseptics and disinfectants due to its ability to kill infection-causing organisms. The gel of the plant can also be directly applied on wounds, which has almost the same effect as an antiseptic medicine. It is therefore especially beneficial in healing open wounds and treating candida.

With anti-fungal and anti-microbial properties, aloe vera extracts come in handy in reducing the growth of dandruff and several skin infections, mainly caused by fungi. It also acts as an antibiotic, having both germicidal and anti-viral medicinal properties.

Aloe Vera eases muscle and joint pain

Did you know aloe vera also helps ease joint pain? Benefits of aloe vera, let me tell you! Aloe vera due to its anti-inflammatory properties provides great relief to those suffering from arthritis, a condition affecting joints and muscles. You can either apply the gel on affected areas or drink aloe juice to reduce pain in joints and muscles. The complex sugars in aloe boost the healing process and provide relief from pain.

Historically Used to Treat Problems from A-Z

In the previous chapters we had a detailed look at the several effective ways in which aloe vera was used by previous generations to keep diseases at bay and lead a healthy life. The benefits of aloe vera are countless; there is hardly any condition that aloe vera cannot provide relief for. You were able to learn about ten benefits of aloe vera, but we still have a lot more to share with you! Here are other health challenges to which aloe vera has been offering solutions since time immemorial.

This list features health benefits for health challenges from A to Z (yes, actually A to Z!)

A – Aloe vera offers protection from allergies, helps with acne, aids acid indigestion, heals abrasions, is effective in managing asthma, athlete's foot, arthritis and also helps to certain extent with AIDS treatment. It also provides relief to those suffering from anemia and arterial insufficiency. However, the extent to which aloe vera can help in treating AIDS is not yet fully known.

B – Burns, bruises, blisters, blemishes, boils and bites are some problems that can be taken care of by using aloe vera. Apart from being a body cleanser, aloe vera also helps with bad breath and those who are bald. It reduces blood pressure and protects the body from bladder infections. It is also helpful in treating bronchitis and bowel irregularity.

C – Candida infections, cold sores, colds, coughs and constipation can be relieved by using aloe vera. It is also helpful in dealing with corneal ulcers, cataract, cystitis and balancing cholesterol level. Aloe vera has also been suggested for cancer treatment. Then it hydrates chapped lips as well as dry skin. However, the effectiveness of aloe vera in treating cancer has not been proven yet.

D – Aloe vera helps in managing diabetes. It is effective in preventing dandruff and moisturizes dry skin, making it healthy. It is also helpful in reducing the pain caused by denture sores, diaper rash, and is also effective against dysentery.

E – Eczema, earache and edema are health conditions that aloe vera provides relief from. It is also helpful in keeping exanthema, erysipelas and epidermitis under control. Aloe vera also fights the Epstein-Barr virus.

F – Aloe vera helps with fungal infections, feline leukemia (FeLV), fibromyalgia and fever.

G – Glaucoma, gingivitis, gassy stomach pain and genital herpes are some of the health conditions for which aloe vera provides relief.

H – Headache relief, heartburn, heat rash, keeping high blood pressure under control, haemorrhoids and herpes are some more problems that aloe vera takes care of.

I – Aloe vera helps with reducing the pain and symptoms from inflamed joints (or any kind of inflammation), insomnia, infertility (if it is caused by anovulatory cycles), insect bites, impetigo, ingrown toenails, indigestion and interstitial cystitis.

J – Aloe vera is helpful in treating jaundice while also easing joint pain.

K – The miracle plant supports treatment and prevention of infections in the kidney and relieves pain caused by keratosis follicularis, which is an inherited skin condition that leads to formation of lesions (similar to warts) on the skin.

L – Aloe vera aids treatment of leprosy, liver problems and laryngitis. Aloe vera juice is also said to stop the development of leukemia cells in the body and helps with lactation for nursing mothers.

M – Muscle cramps, mouth irritation and multiple sclerosis are some more conditions that can be controlled with aloe vera. It is also helpful in preventing and treating mastitis in cattle.

N – Aloe vera is helpful in relieving nausea.

O – Oral problems like bad breath, gingivitis and denture sores can be solved with aloe vera. It also helps in controlling the odour caused by chronic ulcers, as well as boosting onycholysis treatment.

P – Aloe vera helps reduce pain in the pelvis. It is also useful in treating pinworms, prostatitis and psoriasis. It even supports pancreas in insulin production, thereby helping diabetics in managing the condition.

R – Aloe vera is used to treat rashes, radiation-induced burns and razor burns.

S – Aloe vera comes in handy when treating sunburns. It is also effective in fading stretch marks. It is used to treat staph infections, sprains and stings. Also helpful in reducing sores, silicon toxicity, seborrhea and sickle cell disease.

T – Aloe vera is recommended when treating tuberculosis, tendinitis and tonsillitis. It is also said to have a shrinking effect on tumors.

U – Aloe vera is used for treating ulcers – both duodenal and peptic. Also recommended for reducing the symptoms of urticaria, popularly know as hives.

V – The wonder plant is also beneficial in treating venereal sores and varicose veins. Venous stasis is a condition wherein veins (in the legs) lose their ability to carry blood to the heart. The healing and anti-inflammatory properties of aloe vera are also put to use when treating vaginitis.

W – Aloe vera is helpful in treating warts and healing wounds (of any kind). It also helps with windburn.

X – Aloe vera helps soothe X-ray burns.

Y – Yeast infections can be treated with aloe vera.

Z – Aloe vera is also helpful in treating zoster, which is a painful skin rash caused by the same virus that is responsible for spreading chickenpox.

That's not all, folks! These are just the health benefits of aloe vera. Don't you want to know how aloe vera can give you glowing skin and lustrous hair? Learn all that and much more in the next chapter!

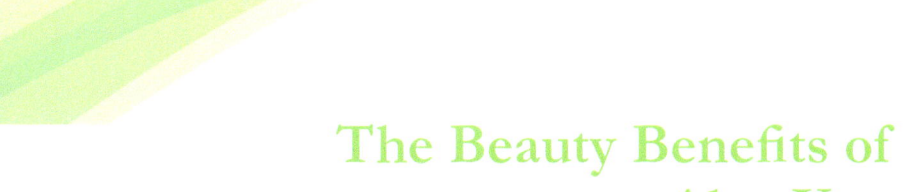

The Beauty Benefits of
Aloe Vera

Aloe vera is a plant that is found in dry arid regions around the world, including Africa, Europe, Asia and the Americas. It is a succulent plant that is frequently grown as an ornamental plant. Its botanical name is *Aloe barbadensis miller* and it belongs to the lily and onion family of plants. The plant is known for its many health benefits and has been used for medicinal purposes by cultures around the world for centuries.

Aloe vera has a number of active ingredients that make it healthy and useful for a number of medicinal purposes.

Vitamins – Vitamins A, C, E, B12, along with choline and folic acid, are present in this plant. It has antioxidant properties that neutralize free radicals in the body that cause aging.

Minerals – It contains copper, magnesium, calcium, chromium, manganese, potassium, zinc, selenium and sodium. These help maintain the metabolic rate of the body; act as antioxidants and help proper functioning of enzymes in the body.

Enzymes – The aloe vera plant contains a number of enzymes, including amylase, cellulose, catalase, alkaline phosphatase, lipase, bradykinase, aliiase, carboxypepditase and peridoxase. They all help break down fats and sugars in the body. Bradykinase also helps reduce excessive skin inflammation.

Fatty acids – Lupeol, beta-sitosterol, cholesterol and campesterol are four plant-based steroids that are found naturally in aloe vera. They have analgesic, antiseptic and anti-inflammatory properties.

Sugars – The plant contains both mono saccharides and polysaccharides. Monosaccharaides such as fructose, monnos-6-phosphate and glucose, along with polysaccharides like glucomannans and polymannose have been found in the gel extract of the aloe vera plant. These are macronutrients required by the body.

Anthraquinones – The aloe vera plant consists of phenolic compounds known for their laxative properties, along with compounds known for their antiviral, analgesic and antibacterial properties.

Amino acids – Each plant contains 7 essential amino acids and 20 of all the amino acids required by the body to function properly. Some of these acids have antiseptic and anti-inflammatory properties.

The giant list of benefits

The benefits of using aloe vera seem almost endless. The gel extracted from the plant can be used for a number of purposes, both medicinal and cosmetic. Here is a list of possible benefits of aloe vera gel, through both topical application and ingestion:

• Treats skin blisters and scarring from minor burns

• Acts as a sun block, relieves irritation from sunburns, and removes an excessive tan

• Relieves skin sensitivity due to frostbite and extreme cold

• Soothes swelling and spots from insect bites on the skin

- Helps alleviate symptoms of allergic skin reactions

- Helps treat rosacea, acne and pimples

- Moisturizes skin to keep it soft and supple

- Works as a scrub and exfoliator to remove dead skin

- Improves hair quality and growth when massaged on to the scalp

- Relieves indigestion, constipation and bloating

- Helps lower blood sugar levels

- Helps control cholesterol levels in the body

- Works as a detoxifier to cleanse the body inside and out for glowing skin and a healthy you.

Heals skin problems

Aloe vera gel is like a magic potion for skin. The gel has many properties that make it an excellent remedy for a number of skin problems, both acute and chronic. Topical application of the gel helps with acute or minor problems like burns and itchiness, while ingestion of the gel can be more helpful for chronic issues like acne and skin infections.

Applying the gel over the burn area for example, can soothe minor burns affecting the first layer of the skin, after touching a hot vessel. For more major burns, it can be mixed with creams or vitamin E.

Applying fresh aloe vera gel to the affected area can treat all acne, pimples, pimple scars, and skin blemishes.

You can get rid of scars due to minor burns, cuts and wounds by applying the gel over the area regularly until the scars disappear.

TIP: Apply on a small area of healthy skin before using to treat skin problems to ensure that you are not allergic to any components in aloe vera gel.

Treats acne and pimples

Pure aloe vera gel is an extremely useful natural remedy in treating acne, drying out pimples and getting rid of acne and pimple scars. It may be used either by itself or in combination with other treatments, creams and medicines.

Depending on how old and how deep your scars are, it can take anywhere between a few weeks to a few months for the scars to disappear completely. It is important to be regular with your application of aloe vera gel. You can safely leave the gel on your skin for hours.

It is important to use pure aloe vera gel for any kind of topical application to ensure maximum benefit. The best way is to either grow an aloe vera plant at home, or to buy full leaves and extract the gel yourself just before applying. If this is not possible, you can look for 100 percent aloe gel products that do not have added chemicals or fragrance.

Lightens skin tone, improves complexion

Aloe vera extract is known to help improve the complexion. The gel extracted from the plant can be used to help make the skin look and feel better. Aloe vera gel helps the skin in many ways, resulting in a fairer, clearer complexion.

It helps fade scars from acne, pimples and wounds. It can also help treat acne and pimples.

• It helps prevent sunburn and if you get a sunburn, it helps soothe the skin and heal it faster.

• It acts as a sunblock and prevents an excessive tan.

• It can be used as a body scrub to get rid of dust, dirt and dead cells from the skins surface.

• It acts as a moisturizer when applied daily, and helps keep the skin smooth, soft and supple.

All of these benefits together help improve your skin's complexion and makes you look and feel younger. The natural plant extract with medicinal value is only effective, if used on a regular basis.

Reduces inflammation and redness

Aloe vera gel has a number of components that are known for their anti-inflammatory properties. These components work together to relieve itchiness, irritation and inflammation of the skin. When they reduce inflammation, the redness is reduced and this makes the skin look and feel more normal.

Since aloe vera gel is a natural plant extract, it does not have side effects on most people. Although, it is better to do a patch test the very first time you use pure aloe vera extract to ensure you are not allergic to any of its components.

Aloe vera gel is soothing to the skin, it relieves redness and inflammation, cools the surface of the skin and helps keep the skin hydrated reducing irritation and dryness. If it is a mild inflammation, the gel can help you feel immediate relief. Remember that inflammation and redness are only symptoms and you have to take care of the root cause of the problem for long-term relief.

Treats sunburns, reduces stretch marks

Stretch marks can appear on various parts of the body due to numerous reasons:

- Puberty

- Sudden or excessive weight gain

- Pregnancy

- Excessive use of topical steroid creams

They may also appear due to a variety of genetic and other health disorders.

Sunburns, on the other hand, are caused by continued exposure to harsh sunlight. Sunburns affects the epidermis, or the outer layer of the skin, stretch marks are caused by scarring of the dermis, or the inner layer of the skin which can be seen from the outside. Aloe vera extract can help soothe sunburned skin by helping cool it down and hydrating it. It also helps the skin heal better without making it too dry and itchy. In the case of stretch marks, since they are found deeper in the skin, regular applications of gel can help fade out the marks over time and make the skin appear more even toned.

Improves skin firmness

As you age, your skin will start sagging and you may lose the firmness and the sculpted look that you had when you were younger. This can happen on your face, as well as the skin on the rest of the body. If there is a lot of sagging, it may change the way clothes fit you. Sagging is a natural process that can take place even if you exercise regularly and maintain a good fitness level. Some people are also more genetically inclined to wrinkle and sag.

If you are looking for natural remedies for sagging skin, one that does not have any side effects with topical application, then you should consider trying aloe vera gel extract. The gel is known to boost the skin's collagen production. Collagen is a natural protein that helps keep the skin tight and firm. Ensure you are not allergic to the extract before applying on larger areas of the skin.

Natural moisturizer for dry skin (makes feet baby soft)

Dry skin can be caused by a variety of reasons. You could naturally have dry skin, or dryness due to a sudden change in climate, a skin infection like eczema or psoriasis, be responding to sun and wind, among other reasons. It can, therefore, be a natural state of your skin, or a symptom or side effect of an infection or disorder.

Aloe vera can help treat dryness of the skin, irrespective of whether it is a symptom or just the way your skin is. If the dryness of your skin is a symptom, aloe vera can help alleviate the dryness until the root cause of the dryness is treated and cured. If it is the way your skin naturally is, it can help hydrate and moisturize it, so that it stays supple and soft.

If you have dry, cracked heels, aloe vera can also work wonders to heal the cracks and make your feet look great and feel baby soft.

Prevents dark circles under the eyes

Dark circles under the eyes are quite common, and are mostly seen in adults of all ages and sexes. There are a number of reasons why dark circles may appear. They may be hereditary, especially if seen in kids. Other reasons include sleep deprivation, excessive sleep, anemia, stress, black eyes, exposure to harsh sunlight, skin pigmentation problems, allergies and thinning of the skin under the eyes with age, among other things. If it is hereditary, there is not much you can do to treat dark circles for good, because dark circles might reappear at any point. But if it is due to one of the other reasons, changes in lifestyle, along with the use of aloe vera extract can help fade away dark circles.

Aloe vera contains vitamins that help improve the elasticity of the skin and get rid of excessive melanin. These vitamins are also key ingredients in many under eye creams, and they can help reduce and get rid of dark circles and wrinkles under the eyes in no time.

Heals swollen lips

There are a number of reasons for you to develop swelling in your lips. Lips swell up when there is excessive build-up of fluid in the area, or when the lips are inflamed. There are many reasons for swollen lips, an allergic reaction being the most common cause. Physical impact and injury, insect bites, sunburn, dehydration and excessive chafing of the lips can also cause them to swell. Certain medical conditions and medicines can also cause lips to swell up.

Aloe vera extract contains many components that are known for their anti-inflammatory properties. Pure aloe vera extract (juice, skin or gel) can be applied directly onto swollen lips and left to dry. Since it is a natural remedy without added chemicals, it can be left on for long hours or even overnight without any problems.

The aloe vera extract reduces swelling by reducing inflammation in the lips and soothing the skin. If the swelling is due to an underlying condition, this will need to be treated to avoid recurrence.

Prevents frequent hair loss

Hair loss is a problem that people of all ages and both sexes have to deal with. It can occur at any age and may be permanent. Major causes of excessive and frequent hair loss are stress, hormonal changes and imbalance, protein deficiency, dandruff, sudden loss of weight, excessive use of styling products and treatments, aging, cancer treatment and excessive use of steroids. It can also be hereditary.

If you are experiencing excessive hair loss, aloe vera extract might be helpful. Aloe vera has active components that are soothing to the skin. The extract is also good for hydration of the scalp. Using aloe vera regularly on the scalp helps reduce dryness, inflammation and itchiness, helps keep the scalp moisturized, cools the skin down, and provides hair follicles with nutrients to make them healthy and strong. All this together can help reduce thinning or excessive hair loss and make your hair look and feel healthy, strong and lustrous.

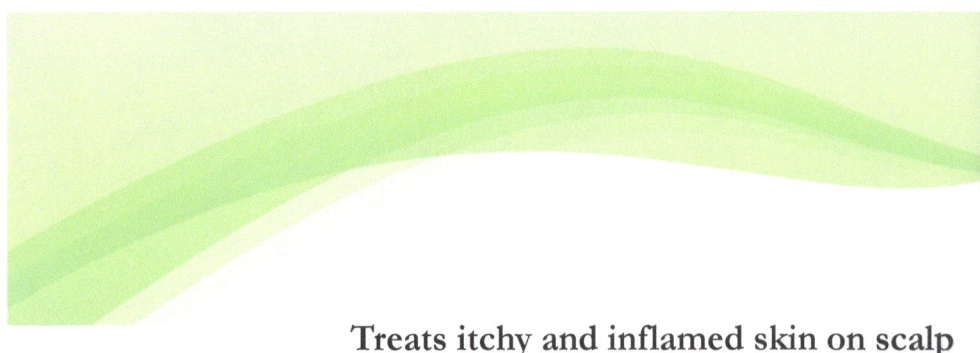

Treats itchy and inflamed skin on scalp

The scalp is one part of the body that is not exposed to sunlight or the elements as much as other parts of the body, because it is usually covered by hair. Your scalp can be more sensitive to external and internal changes, becoming irritated and inflamed due various reasons. Dandruff, clogging of pores due to excessive secretion of oil, heat and sweat, dehydration or itchiness can cause the skin of the scalp to become inflamed and irritated.

Aloe vera gel and extract has a number of active ingredients that are known for their anti-inflammatory properties. Using aloe vera extract for topical application regularly can help reduce inflammation, dryness and relieve itchiness of the scalp.

You can massage aloe vera juice or gel directly on to the scalp. Apply the extract and slowly massage it into the scalp using the tips of your fingers. You should be gentle and not apply too much pressure when massaging. Of course, if you can find someone to help you with this step, even better!

Treats and prevents dandruff

Dandruff is a very common problem faced by people everywhere. Some common causes of dandruff include dryness of the scalp, fungal infections, dry climate, excessive or diminished secretion of skin oils, among other things. Stress and nutritional deficiencies can further aggravate the incidence and severity of dandruff. The scalp may feel inflamed if there is excessive itchiness and irritation of the scalp. Although it is not harmful in any way, it can be irritating and itchy, causing it to be an embarrassing distraction at times, especially in public.

If you are constantly faced with dandruff problems, aloe vera might be a good remedy that you could try. Aloe vera extract is known for its anti-inflammatory properties that can help soothe the scalp. It helps hydrate the skin and reduces itchiness and irritation due to excessive dryness. It also helps reduce fungal growth and excessive secretion of skin oils, which can in turn help reduce dandruff.

Acts as natural hair conditioner

Most people who have even slightly longer hair will understand the pain of managing hair and making it look good every day. Hair can get frizzy and unmanageable if there is too much dust and pollution, if it is too windy or if the climate is dry. Hair also dries out due to dehydration, dandruff and lack of adequate secretion of skin oils in the scalp. Dry hair is difficult to manage, and gets knotted easily, making you look scruffy and disheveled. If your hair dries out very often and you like conditioner, or if you have not found a conditioner that really helps condition and manage your hair, you could consider trying aloe vera.

Aloe vera extract is a great way to hydrate the hair naturally. The extract also contains vitamins that can nourish the hair and make it healthier. Better hydration and nourishment helps naturally condition the hair and make it look lustrous and feel healthy.

Restores hair's natural strength and beauty

If your scalp is not adequately hydrated, your hair can appear dry. Dandruff, excessive or inadequate oil secretion, dust, pollution, sweat and changes in climate can have a negative affect on your hair. Nutritional deficiencies and stress can also contribute to a decline in scalp and hair health. Your hair may end up looking dull and lifeless, and may become weak and brittle over time. How do you restore hair and scalp health using natural remedies? Aloe vera extract is a great natural remedy to treat dull, lifeless hair. The extract is extremely hydrating to the scalp and to the hair shaft. Better hydration means that your hair will be more bouncy and smooth. The extract also has anti-inflammatory properties that can help soothe the scalp and reduce itchiness and dandruff. It also contains vitamins and minerals essential for good scalp and hair health.

Massage aloe vera extract onto the scalp regularly, or use it as a conditioner to make your hair look amazing and feel healthy.

Acts as a perfect hair rinse

Sometimes washing your hair leaves a lot to be desired. It can leave your hair dry, knotted, frizzy and impossible to manage. Shampooing can also strip the hair and scalp of essential skin oils to keep the scalp and hair shafts hydrated and soft. If you do not use the right conditioner, these problems will persist and affect the way your hair looks and feels.

If you are looking for a hair rinse that will help hydrate, moisturize and soften your hair, then aloe vera extract is worth a try. The extract is extremely hydrating and nourishing for the hair. Also, since it is a natural extract with no added chemicals, you can rinse your hair with it and leave it on the hair all day without any problems. It forms a protective layer on hair shafts and keeps dust and pollution at bay, while keeping the scalp hydrated, nourished and cool.

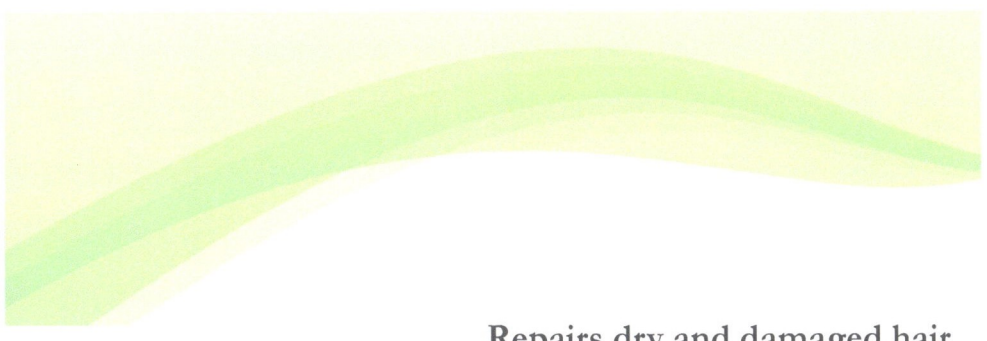

Repairs dry and damaged hair

Hair is sensitive to internal changes in the body and external changes in the environment. If there is any imbalance or sudden change in either internal or external conditions, it can cause damage to the hair and can make it look dry, dull and lifeless. Dry climate, excessive exposure to harsh sunlight, dehydration, nutritional deficiencies and stress can all contribute to poor hair health. Swimming frequently in chlorinated water can strip the hair of essential oils and make it look dull & lifeless, too.

Aloe vera extract can help protect your hair against external environmental factors and can also help with certain internal factors as well. The extract helps hydrate the hair shafts and scalp, and provides essential vitamins and minerals to keep the hair healthy. Using it as a conditioner or a rinse after shampooing creates a protective layer on the hair. This helps keep the scalp cool, while protecting hair from dust and pollution.

Treats Alopecia

Alopecia is a medical condition where the immune system of the body attacks hair follicles like it would attack infections in the body. This results in sudden loss of hair, bald patches and excessive hair loss over time. Young adults and teenagers are more frequently affected by alopecia, although it could affect people of other ages as well. Alopecia areata results in sudden hair loss, while alopecia androgenetica refers to male pattern baldness and is a slower process. Aloe vera contains components that are known to help balance and normalize the functioning of the immune system.

Massaging it into the scalp can help prevent the immune system from attacking hair follicles and causing your hair to fall out. The extract also contains a number of active ingredients and nutrients that can restore scalp and hair health. This can help your hair grow back faster once the alopecia has been treated. It can also ensure that hair becomes healthier, less brittle and more lustrous.

The Wellness Benefits of Aloe Vera

Introduction

Most people associate aloe vera with simple topical applications, such as healing for sunburned skin, or acne scars, but aloe vera has properties that go beyond these uses. Most people are also aware that it can be beneficial for minor burns, wounds, scars, hair loss, dandruff, general cleansing, exfoliation, inflammation and redness, moisturization and such other similar uses. It is known to soothe the skin, and helps keep the skin hydrated and supple.

However, what most people do not know is that aloe vera can also be consumed. There are a few species of aloe vera that can be ingested safely, without any toxic side effects. But why would you consume aloe vera? The answer is that aloe vera extract,usually found in a juicy gel form, contains a number of macro and micro nutrients that are essential for the body to function optimally.

Aloe vera extract contains vitamins, minerals, amino acids, sugars and other nutrients, along with enzymes and anthraquinones. These active ingredients help not only keep the skin and body healthy, but are also known to improve brain function, and boost immunity.

Just under the green outer layer of the aloe vera leaves, there is a translucent gel-like substance that is found in each plant. This gel can simply be squeezed out or cut out with the help of a normal kitchen knife. It is a little slimy and slippery to touch and could have a slightly bitter aftertaste. The green part of the leaves contains juice, which can be squeezed out by pressing on the inner surface of the leaf once the gel has been removed.

Here are some surprising and amazing ways aloe vera can help you stay healthy and fit in body and mind.

Weight loss

Obesity is one of the biggest problems in the world today. It can cause a number of health problems, such as knee and hip pain, diabetes, cholesterol, blockages in arteries, breathlessness, mobility problems and a general dip in self-confidence. Although a good number of people who are obese have the problem because of wrong lifestyles or making poor diet choices, or other choices that are within their means, that is not the only reason people gain weight. A number of medical conditions, treatments and medicines can also cause sudden and excessive weight gain.

Whatever the cause, it is always a huge challenge to be able to lose weight that you have gained over months and years, and to keep it at a healthy level after you manage to lose the excess weight. People are ready to go on extreme diets and undergo drastic surgeries, putting their health at risk with weight loss procedures that have not been tested or even proven to be helpful.

What if there was a remedy and a way to lose weight naturally without much or almost any side effects and without having to compromise on health even more due to drastic weight loss procedures? There is a natural remedy, one that has been used for centuries by civilizations all over the world, which can aid in healthy weight loss – aloe vera.

How aloe vera helps with weight loss:

1.   It increases the rate of metabolism of the body, so that fats and carbohydrates are burned faster and better, and are not stored in the body as much.

2.   It contains collagen, an essential protein for muscle building. The body spends a considerable amount of energy to assimilate collagen into the body. It, therefore, helps improve muscle tone while losing weight.

3.   It contains essential vitamins & minerals that help speed up metabolism, improves absorption of nutrients and enhances the functioning of digestive glands in the body.

4.   It has laxative properties that help improve bowel movements, so that you will not have problems like constipation, indigestion and bloating.

5.   It helps with better absorption and digestion of sugar. This not only helps control blood sugar level, but also helps you feel full longer, so that you end up eating less.

If you intend to consume aloe vera, ensure that you do your research and get only the kind that is edible. You can use any aloe vera extract for topical applications.

You can consume the gel directly, blended with honey and lemon juice, or mixed with other vegetable or fruit juices. Ensure that you have it fresh and right after extracting it from the leaf if you are using it directly from the plant. Right before meals or right after waking up in the morning are the best times to consume aloe vera for best results.

Aloe vera is a plant that looks like a cactus but is actually a succulent plant that is part of the liliaceae family of plants. There are over 200 species of aloe vera. They all look similar, but have differing properties, taste and active ingredients, although the general properties and components remain more or less the same. There are less than 10 species of aloe vera that are fit for human consumption. Aloe vera gel is considered to be the best for both consumption and application.

Physical fitness

The burning of sugars, carbohydrates and fats in the body produces energy. The more these nutrients are burned, the more energy is produced. There are many reasons like aging, medical conditions, stress and obesity that can cause a drop in the level of energy you have for day-to-day activates.

Aloe vera has active ingredients that help increase the metabolic rate of your body. Increased metabolism means that your body produces more energy and you will then feel more alive and active throughout the day. Aloe vera also helps relieve stress, reduces weight and alleviates symptoms of various medical conditions that may be pulling your energy levels down. It, therefore, increases vitality and you feel more vibrant and energetic throughout the day and do not tire so easily.

Detoxification

Detoxification refers to cleansing the body of unwanted chemicals and substances that can be harmful. Detoxification helps rid the body of excessive alcohol & drugs, cholesterol & toxic waste produced by the body. It also cleans the liver, the lymphatic system and blood, and helps control acid reflux, indigestion and constipation, among other things. A good detox can give you healthy glowing skin and lustrous hair.

Aloe vera works really well as a detox. The plant extract contains essential vitamins and minerals, as well as a number of enzymes and collagen, all of which come together to help cleanse the body from the inside to give you soft skin, a healthy body and glossy hair. The extract has a mild laxative effect that ensures good bowel movements and reduces the instances of bloating, constipation and indigestion. It also helps improve immunity so you are less prone to common infections.

Anti-aging

Aging is a natural process that causes a number of changes in the body. It can cause wrinkles, sagging skin, reduced muscle tone, and can change your entire body structure. Wrinkling and sagging skin can make you appear older than you are, give you a jowl and take away the sculpted look of your face and body.

Aloe vera can help reduce the appearance of wrinkles, fine lines, reduce sagging of skin and loosening of muscles. It contains vitamins A, B12, C and E along with choline and folic acid, all of which help fight free radicals in the body. Free radicals are the chemicals that cause signs of aging to appear on the skin.

Aloe vera also contains collagen, which is an essential protein in muscle building. Collagen helps tighten and plump up the skin to make it firmer and reduce sagging by improving overall muscle tone of the body.

Adaptogen

An adaptogen is a natural substance, usually a herb, which has the ability to work positively on the human body and improve functioning of all the vital systems and organs of the body without any long lasting or drastic side effects. Aloe vera has been classified as an adaptogen because of its ability to help the human body function well without long-term side effects.

- Control blood sugar levels.

- Boost the immune system.

- Keep the brain healthy.

- Keep the heart and arteries free of cholesterol build-up.

- Ensure proper functioning of various glands of the body.

Since it is able to benefit the various body systems positively without any drastic side effects, it is very popular for topical applications and for consumption all over the world. Being an adaptogen makes it ideal for various medicinal and cosmetic uses.

Reduces stress, increases well-being

Stress is one of the leading causes of many acute and chronic health problems that people suffer from today. It can cause hypertension, diabetes, muscle aches, migraines, hair loss, and flare up thyroid issues. Long hours at work, managing the house single-handedly, and having small kids to take care of can stress you out by the end of the day. It is important to be able to relax and rid yourself of aches and pains at the end of each day so you can sleep well and start every day fresh and rejuvenated.

You can freeze aloe vera extract to make ice cubes. The extract has a lot of water content, which makes it easy to freeze. You can, alternatively, add the extract to ice trays with water and freeze this instead. These ice cubes can be used as a cold compress or just to massage your forehead and shoulders after a long day at work. The cold helps relax sore muscles, and the aloe vera helps hydrate, soothe and reduce inflammation and pain.

How to Incorporate Aloe Vera into Your Life

Aloe vera is considered by many to be a magic potion of sorts, a plant with an unbelievable number of benefits. It has both cosmetic and medicinal value. Its extracts can be found in the form of juice and gel. It can be bought as a pure extract, or combined with creams and lotions which have pure aloe extract in them. It can help remove scars, reduce dandruff, hydrate skin, improve bowel movement, cleanse the blood, increase immunity, soothe burns and inflammation, among many other uses.

If you are a fan of aloe vera and its natural health benefits, but are wondering how to incorporate it into everyday life, here are a few ways that you can make aloe vera an intrinsic part of your daily beauty and health regimen with ease.

As a makeup remover

Makeup removers usually contain a lot of oils, which may clog pores as you remove your makeup. Sensitive areas like the skin around the eyes and lips can have breakouts and acne if removers are too heavy on oils.

If you want something more gentle and natural, use aloe vera extract. Apply the extract around your eyes with a cotton ball and slowly wipe it off as it dries. It will remove all your makeup, cleanse and hydrate your skin, leaving you with soft supple skin that is unclogged and clean.

As night cream

Night creams are meant to be mild because they are left on the skin overnight. They are usually meant for the face, which has thinner and more sensitive skin than the rest of the body. But most night creams come with fragrance or unwanted chemicals that may do your skin more harm than good.

You can use aloe vera extract instead of your regular night cream. You can rub the skin, or the gel onto your face, or mix it in with your regular night cream. Aloe vera extract helps hydrate the skin, removes scars and keeps your skin soft and supple. It can also help you avoid early sagging & reduce wrinkles; leaving your skin firm and glowing every morning.

As shaving cream

Most shaving creams have a lot of synthetic chemicals and additives that can harm your skin with regular usage. They also dehydrate the skin, leaving it rough and dry after every shave.

Using aloe vera gel for shaving can be beneficial in many ways. It has a smooth slippery texture, so that you can shave easily without forcing the razor to move on your skin and helps you avoid razor burns. Aloe vera gel contains over 90 percent water, which means that it is mild and leaves your skin hydrated after your shave. Ensure you use pure aloe vera gel without any additives.

As burn cream

One of the most well-known uses of aloe vera extract is in the treatment of sunburned skin. When applied on sunburned skin, aloe helps cool and soothe the skin. Because of its hydrating properties, it also softens burned skin, so that there is minimal or no peeling or scarring as the skin heals.

It can also be used to treat minor burns from matches and after touching hot vessels. It soothes burned inflamed skin, prevents excessive blistering and helps the skin heal faster. It has antiseptic properties as well, which prevent infection on burn wounds. It also helps remove scars from minor burns and reduce the effects of excessive tanning.

As soothing ice cube

You can freeze aloe vera extract into ice cubes. These ice cubes can be used when you want to cool and hydrate your skin. They are relaxing to muscles and skin after a long hard day. These cubes can also be used to relax tired eyes, especially if you work long hours staring into a computer and other digital devices. They are great to cleanse the skin after being out in dust and pollution. Slowly massage your skin with these ice cubes in a circular motion for best results.

As face wash or mouth wash

Active ingredients in aloe vera have antibacterial, antiseptic and anti-inflammatory properties. When aloe vera extract is used as a face wash, it not only helps cleanse the skin and clear pores, but also ensures that you do not have a breakout of acne and pimples. It also soothes and hydrates the skin, so that your face feels clean, smooth and soft after you wash it with the extract.

Because of its antiseptic and antibacterial properties, along with analgesic properties, aloe vera extract works really well as a mouthwash. It reaches all corners of the mouth where you are unable to brush, cleans teeth, gums and empty tooth sockets, reduces pain from infections or tooth extractions and keeps oral infections away.

As hand sanitizer

The main function of hand sanitizers is to kill bacteria, viruses and other germs that may make you unwell or cause infections in the body. Most sanitizers achieve this by adding alcohol to the mix. Alcohol works well to sterilize and kill bacteria, but it also dries out the hands. Sanitizers also have a lot of unwanted chemicals that can harm you if ingested regularly.

Instead, you can carry a small bottle of pure aloe vera extract with you wherever you go. Using this extract as a hand sanitizer not only gets rid of infection-causing germs, but also leaves your hands moisturized and hydrated. It is also safe to be ingested on a regular basis.

As juice to reduce blood sugar, cholesterol and triglycerides

The juice of aloe vera is extracted from the green skin of the leaves, and blended along with the gel extracted from the plant leaves. The juice is very watery and translucent in color. It feels almost like water, but has a slightly slippery texture and a mild bitter aftertaste.

This juice is known to help control blood sugar levels by helping the cells absorb sugar better. It also has a cleansing effect, cleaning the blood and lymphatic system from toxins and impurities, which include cholesterol and triglyceride deposits in the artery walls. This prevents artery walls from hardening and arteries from getting clogged.

As detox, or body cleanse juice

Aloe vera is known to have mild laxative properties. Although it is not healthy to be dependent on laxatives, you can use the extract every once in a while to keep your bowel movements normal, or if you have a bout of indigestion, constipation or bloating. If the problem persists after a few days of aloe vera usage, consult your doctor who can then search for underlying health problems.

It can also be used for a detox routine for a general body cleansing every few months. You can add it to smoothies or vegetable & fruit juices a few times a week. If you are all right with its texture and taste, you can also consume the juice or gel directly or with a bit of honey. It can be mixed with lime juice, honey and water for the ultimate detox, preferably first thing in the morning.

Five Tips for Using Aloe Vera

At this point, you should be aware of the unlimited benefits of aloe vera, be it for your health, skin or wellness. In this chapter, we will shed light on some more (five to be precise) ways in which you can include aloe vera in your diet, skincare regime and even weight loss program!

Making aloe vera juice at home

You already know about the benefits of drinking aloe vera juice. It is natural and cleans your body from within. It boosts your energy levels by flushing toxins out of your body. What if we told you that you could make this miracle energy drink at home? Yes, you can make aloe vera juice in your very own kitchen.

•   Get one Aloe Barbadensis Miller plant leaf, wash it and cut its outer green cover with a knife.

•   Next take off the sap, the yellow slimy layer covering the gel. You should peel away about one to two millimetres of the skin of the leaf to get to the gel.

•   Take out the gel from the leaf, as needed. It should be clear, without any sap sticking to it. You can also use a spoon to scrape it out.

•   Place the gel in a blender immediately and mix it until you get a smooth paste.

•   Mix two tablespoons of the aloe gel with 250 ml water to make one glass of aloe vera juice. Your all-natural, healthy aloe vera juice is ready!

Alternately, you can add some flavor to your juice by blending two tablespoons of the gel with one cup of orange or grapefruit juice (you could use any citrus-based juice). Make sure that you store the remaining aloe vera gel in the refrigerator. You can have the drink once either in the morning (at least 30 minutes before having your breakfast) or in the evening, three hours before sleeping. If you take any sort of medication, discuss the idea of adding aloe vera in your diet with your doctor or naturopath before going ahead with it.

How to make an aloe skin mask

Aloe vera benefits your skin in more ways than one and you are going to love how it gives your skin a healthy glow. There are several ways to treat your skin with an aloe mask. The simplest way is to just rub aloe vera gel on your face, while other methods involve combining a few natural ingredients with the gel. Here we share some of the easiest and most effective ones:

Aloe vera and lemon mask

This mask is excellent for those with oily or acne prone skin as both aloe vera and lemon work miraculously to fade acne marks and blemishes. Blend aloe vera gel (we have already explained to you how to separate the gel from the leaf) with the juice from half a lemon, and that's all - your aloe vera-lemon mask is ready! Apply the mixture to your face and wash it off after 15 minutes. Do it regularly, (once or twice a week) to see your acne marks fading and your skin getting lighter.

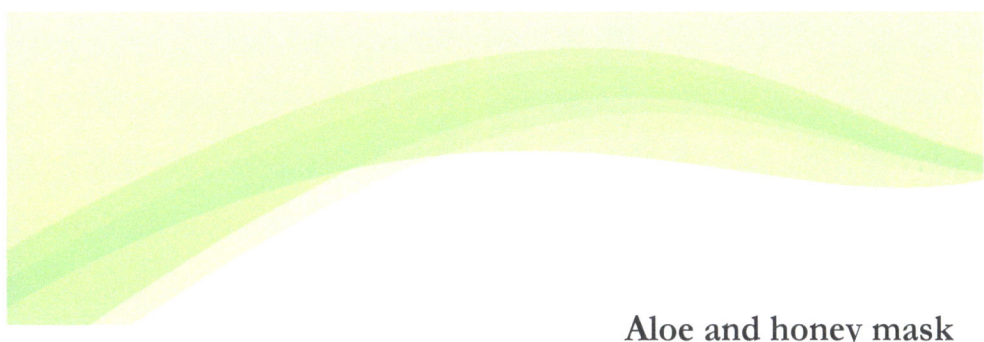

Aloe and honey mask

Just like aloe vera, honey too is known for its anti-septic properties and is effective in clearing marks and blemishes from the skin. It makes for a soothing mask and are the instructions:

Mix one tablespoon of honey and aloe vera gel (blend it into a paste so that it is easier to mix and apply). After both the ingredients have been mixed thoroughly, apply the mask on your face and leave it on for 20 minutes before washing it in warm water.

Aloe, sugar and milk

Combine aloe, sugar and milk to treat your skin with an exfoliating mask that will get rid of all dead skin and blackheads. Mix one-tablespoon sugar, half a tablespoon of milk and two tablespoons of aloe vera gel. This can be made at home or you can use any natural store-bought variety. If you have an aloe vera tree plant, make sure you carefully scrape out the sap sticking to the gel before adding to the blender to make a paste. Leave the mask on your face for 20 minutes and then wash it off. Sugar will exfoliate your skin, milk will moisten & tone it, while aloe vera will soothe & brighten it.

Anti-aging aloe yoghurt mask

Make the best use of the anti-aging properties of aloe vera by mixing it with yoghurt, which has a cooling effect on the skin. Mix two tablespoons of aloe gel with one-tablespoon honey and two tablespoons of fresh yoghurt. Cover both your face and neck with the cooling mask and relax for 30 minutes. Wash it off to reveal fresh and radiant skin. It is recommended for those dealing with aging problems like wrinkles, fine lines and age spots.

Storing aloe vera at home

Got a noticeable suntan? Aloe vera can help you with it. Need a soothing face cream? Ditch that chemical-filled face serum and use some aloe vera gel instead. The same goes for when you need to style your hair, a little aloe vera gel and your hairstyle will stay in place. Isn't it amazing how one plant can offer so many benefits? It's a great habit to rely on aloe vera for almost any of your problems – be it weight loss or skin care. So did you just blend some aloe vera gel to make a detox drink and are now wondering what to do with the remaining gel? You don't have to worry about it going bad, you can store the gel in your refrigerator for 8-10 days. To make it last a little longer (and give it a refreshing, citrus scent), you can add some drops of lemon juice to the gel. How about aloe vera gel cubes? They last long and add a twist to your regular ice cubes – all you have to do it freeze the gel in ice cube bags or trays and pop them out whenever you need them.

What if we told you your stored aloe vera gel could last last as long as 6-8 months? Here is the secret – break open Vitamin C or E capsules (0.2 percent) and add it to fresh aloe vera gel in a blender. This simple trick will ensure that your aloe vera gel will last without losing its medicinal properties. Another way to get scented and long lasting aloe vera is to mix it with essential oils like lavender or rosemary. However, this method is recommended only when you plan to use the gel externally.

If you want to store an aloe vera leaf instead, refrigerating it will make it last for a few weeks while storing it in an airtight bag or box will keep it fresh for up to half a year! Aloe vera juice on the other hand, should be consumed within one week of refrigeration (if not immediately) to get the most benefit out of it.

How to lose weight using aloe vera

Aloe vera not only comes in handy every time you get a bruise, but is also an effective weight loss booster. Remember in the initial chapters we had a look at some of the components in the aloe vera? Well, most of them also do a great job in boosting weight loss. The anti-oxidants in the plant prevent free radicals from thriving in the body. In fact, it boosts your metabolism and keeps your body mass index (BMI) in check. Aloe vera is filled with collagen and proteins, which are great for those aiming to develop muscles in their body. So forget those crash diets, here is how aloe vera can help you lose weight.

•   Mix a half a glass of aloe vera juice with any other fruit juice (even vegetable juice) of your choice, and there you have a refreshing, tasty drink that promotes weight loss! You can also skip the added juice and just drink aloe vera juice mixed with some water.

•   Mix some fresh aloe vera gel with any flavored juice as a metabolism booster. Alternately, you can also take an aloe vera gel capsule, which has the same effect on the body as the aloe vera juice.

•   Another tasty as well as effective way to lose weight using aloe vera is to blend its gel with some lemon juice. You can also add a drop of honey to add some sweetness to it. Drink any of these concoctions regularly while doing any at least 30 minutes of physical activity like running or aerobics daily to see a quick reduction in your weight.

Final Tip

Don't use DIY aloe vera products. Purchase commercial products created by experts so that you enjoy full benefits

Of course, you can use aloe vera fresh from the plant, but that will call for added precautions to be taken. When you use aloe vera directly from the plant, there is a risk of not cleaning the sap sticking to the gel and consuming it accidentally. The sap acts as an irritant for humans so it is essential that when using aloe vera internally, you consume only the gel or juice (distilled with water or other juices as specified). Also, if the aloe vera is not fresh, chances are that it may have lost its medicinal properties, which may not give you the desired benefits.

By getting aloe vera products from reliable manufacturers, you benefit by using best quality, all-natural aloe vera, which is free from any sort of irritant. What's more, by choosing credible sellers like Accomplish Now, you get to choose from a whole range of high quality, natural aloe vera-based products like juices, detox drinks, our skin care range and many more, which will enable you to lead a healthy lifestyle.

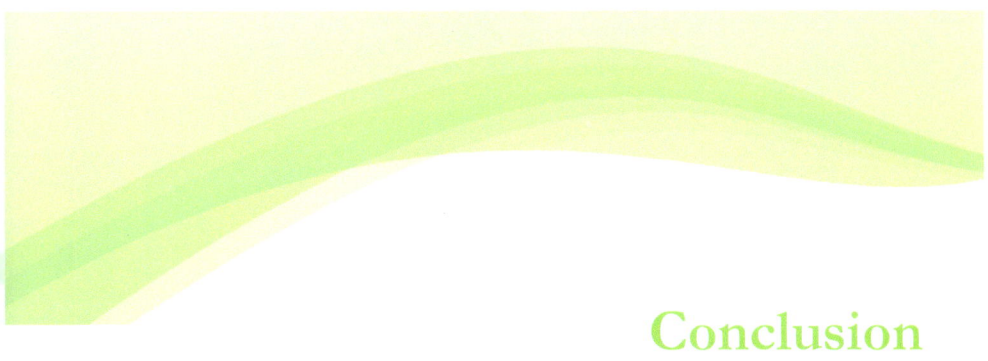

Conclusion

Much before modern technology enabled scientific research by isolating components and understanding atomic and subatomic structures of the plant and its extract, humans knew the benefits of the aloe vera plant. Since ancient Egyptian civilizations 4,000 years ago, aloe vera has been used extensively in traditional medicine and beauty treatments for its myriad health benefits. Science has only now discovered some of the many benefits that aloe vera can have on the human body.

Aloe vera contains over 200 active ingredients, which include vitamins, minerals, proteins, amino acids and other nutrients vital to proper functioning of the body. The plant also has antiseptic, antiviral, antibacterial and anti-inflammatory properties. It also has analgesic properties, which are properties of a painkiller.

Aloe vera extract is available mainly in three different forms:

- Juice, which is extracted from the inner part of the skin of the aloe vera leaves.

- Gel, which is the inner, translucent portion of the leaves.

- Capsules, which contain dried juice or gel extracts.

Aloe vera is also easy to grow in almost any climate, needs minimum looking after, and is one of the few plants where you can easily get the extract at home without using any specialized tools or processes. The gel can simply be scooped out using a spoon or knife once you have sliced the aloe vera leaf. It can then be used like a gel, or blended into a juice. It should ideally be consumed immediately after extraction for maximum benefits. It is also equally easy to incorporate into your daily health and beauty regimen.

Health benefits from aloe vera extract includes better digestive health, improved metabolism & bowel movements, healthy heart & arteries, a cleaner lymphatic system, controlled blood sugar levels, and a stronger immune system.

Beauty benefits of aloe vera extract include reduction of acne and pimples, fading of scars and stretch marks, a clearer complexion, less tanning and burning from exposure to the sun, firmer skin, natural exfoliation and cleansing of the skin, conditioning of hair and treatment of dark circles under the eyes.

Other than all this, it can also provide benefits by reducing wrinkles, and fine lines, detoxifying the body, helping to a great extent with healthy weight loss, reducing stress and effects of stress on the body, and it also works like an adaptogen.

Aloe vera can be easily incorporated into everyday life. For topical applications, it can be used by itself or mixed with your regular lotions and creams. It can be used topically as a shaving gel, moisturizer, aftershave, night cream, face wash, sunblock, as ice cubes, or as a hand sanitizer. For consumption, it can either be directly consumed as a juice or gel, or blended with vegetable and fruit juices, in smoothies, desserts or in lemonade with honey.

As you have seen through this entire book, aloe vera is probably one of the most useful natural sources of medicinal benefits and cosmetic properties today. Its health benefits are innumerable and it is a cost-effective and natural way to look amazing, stay fit and improve overall health and wellness. Say yes to the amazing aloe vera extract and to a healthy natural life.

Contact the person who introduced you to this book. They may know of the right high quality Aloe Vera products and will help you achieve your personal Health, Wellness and Beauty goals!

Your Natural Health, Beauty and Wellness Guide

www.ingramcontent.com/pod-product-compliance
Lightning Source LLC
Chambersburg PA
CBHW050752290526
45792CB00008B/2149